Essential Oils for Dogs
Basic Aromatherapy

Julie Summers

Copyright © 2017 Julie Summers

All rights reserved.

This book is or any part of it may not be reproduced in any written, electronic, recording, or photocopying without written permission of the publisher or author having intellectual rights over the content of the book. The exception would be in the case of brief quotations embodied in the critical articles or reviews and pages where permission is specifically granted by the publisher or author.

Although every precaution has been taken to verify the accuracy of the information contained herein, the author and publisher assume no responsibility for any errors or omissions. No liability is assumed for any damage or damages that may result from the use of information contained herein.

Information contains in this book in solely for information purposes and does not intend in any way to replace professional medical and health advices rendered by practitioners in the field of veterinary medicine and you are further recommended to seek professional advice before using this material.

ISBN-10: 197596182X
ISBN-13: 978-1975961824

CONTENTS

1	INTRODUCTION	1
2	WHAT ARE ESSENTIAL OILS?	3
3	WHAT CAN AROMATHERPY HELP WITH?	10
4	SAFETY MEASURES BEFORE USING ESSENTIAL OILS WITH YOUR DOGS	20
5	IS AROMATHERAPY SUITABLE FOR YOUR DOG?	32
6	DIFFERENT AROMATHERAPY APPLICATIONS	47
7	AROMATHERAPY TOOLS AND MATERIALS	57
8	3 GREAT AROMATHERAPIES FOR YOUR DOG	66

INTRODUCTION

Essential oils have previously been used for enhancement of well-being in humans but, are they safe to use on animals and pets, particularly on dogs that have been proven to be loyal companions of people?

The holistic approach to the use of essential oils for dogs is now gaining popularity among pet and dog lovers but misinformation has also taken its toll on some who were misguided in the proper ways of using essential oils on dogs. Through this eBook, we aim to correct this misinformation and provide you with a safe and easy to follow guide you can use while applying essential oils to your dog.

In this Book, you can expect a thorough

understanding of essential oils on dogs including its various applications, benefits, safety precautions and uses plus, added homemade recipes which are sure to help you minimize your budget while maintaining your dog's health and well-being.

Through this guide, you can provide your pet the essential care he needs to improve his health condition, stabilize his mental and emotional state and improve his behavior.

This holistic approach to aromatherapy is geared towards enhancing the total well-being of your dog and likewise, developing a stronger bond between the two of you.

WHAT ARE ESSENTIAL OILS

An essential oil is an organic compound substance taken from the sac, glandular hair and in any other parts of the plants including leaves, roots, seeds, fruit or flowers. They are the essence of that particular plant and are responsible for the unique scent of that specific plant. An essential oil is volatile and therefore evaporates easily in addition to being diffusible.

Essential oils need to be diluted before each use as they are highly concentrated. Each essential oil carries individual properties like color, scent, healing effects and other chemical properties.

Many of these essential oils are antibacterial,

antifungal, antiviral, antioxidant and anti-inflammatory. They also affect the emotional function of the body by stimulating particular areas of the brain and can even be a sedative.

When you extract essential oils from plants through steam distillation, you can produce hydrosol, a water-based substance, which is a by-product obtained from the initial process. Hydrosol contains only a little part of the essential oil and a large part of the water-soluble parts of the plants. Unlike essential oils which are highly concentrated, hydrosol is not concentrated and can be used undiluted. You can also add essential oils for a combined effect.

For a highly sensitive dog, you can have hydrosol as an alternative option from using essential oils.

How are Essential Oil Made?

To extract a plant's essential oil, you may use the following methods:

- Steam Distillation
- Solvent Extraction
- Carbon Dioxide Extraction
- Manual Extraction

Distillation

The majority of essential oils are produced by the process of distillation. In distillation, water is heated to produce steam, which carries the most volatile substance of the scent. Then the steam is chilled in a condenser and the distilled result is collected. Normally, the essential oil is lighter and so it floats on top of the hydrosol, which is the distilled water component. Later, you will be working on separating the two compound elements.

Steam Distillation

Steam distillation uses an external source of steam, which carries the steam through the pipes into the distillation unit, sometimes at high pressure. Then the steam will pass through the aromatic material and exit into the condenser.

Hydrodistillation

The part of the plant which is used for oil extraction is fully submerged in water, producing the "soup". When steamed, it contains the essential oil or essence. This process is the oldest method and yet the most versatile and is used in primitive countries.

However, there is a risk in this method as the distiller can dry up or overheat giving the essence a burnt smell.

Hydrodistillation works best with powders like spice powders, ground wood and many other tough parts of the plants like the roots as well as other hard materials such as nuts.

Water and Steam Distillation

This method is best for distilling leafy materials but is not applicable for seeds, wood, or roots.

In this method, the leaves are placed in a steamer basket over boiling water, exposing it to the rising steam vapors.

Solvent Extraction

Some flowers used for essential oils like Jasmine and Linden blossom are too delicate to survive the process of distillation. To be able to capture their essence, the process of solvent extraction is used. The blossoms are placed in perforated trays and loaded into an extracting unit. The blossoms are then washed repeatedly using a solvent, usually hexane.

The solution dissolves all the extracted materials which include non-essence wax, highly volatile essential oil and pigments. The solution, with all these dissolvable plant materials and the solvent, is then filtered.

The filtration process is done by subjecting the whole solution to low process distillation to recover the solvent for reuse. The remaining materials that are wax-like are called the concrete and contain as much as 55% of the volatile oil.

To dilute the pure essential oils, it is again processed to remove the wax-like material. To separate the wax; it is warmed and mixed with ethanol alcohol. It is during the heating and stirring process that the concrete is broken up into small globules.

Along with the essence, some wax is also dissolved and can only be removed by freezing the solution at a very low temperature or around 30 degrees Fahrenheit. This way, the wax is separated. As a final precaution, the pure essence is now filtered and declared absolute. This extraction process actually yields three products that you can use. One is the concrete used for solid perfumes, the pure essential oil and the floral waxes which are used as additives to candles, thickening creams and lotions as an alternative to beeswax.

Carbon Dioxide Extraction

When Carbon Dioxide (CO_2) is exposed to high pressure, it changes into liquid form. Its liquid form can be chemically inactive and safe which can then be used to extract the aromatic molecules in a process akin to how the absolutes are extracted. With this process, there will be no traces of solvent residues because CO_2 is again exposed to normal pressure and temperature. It will only revert to its gaseous form and evaporate.

Cold Pressing

Notice that when you score or zest the skin of an orange, you get to see the spray of its essential oil. In the process of cold pressing, machines are able to do just this way. They can mass-produce citrus oils by doing the same procedure—scoring the rinds and capturing the oil that comes out of them. While citrus oils can also be produced through the steam distillation process, the result seems to be of lower quality compared to the ones produced by cold pressing.

Florasols or Phytonic Process

Florasol or phytol process is the newest method used in extracting essential oils by utilizing non-CFS (non-chlorofluorocarbons) as solvents. The oils are called phytols, hence the name of the method it stands for. The unique properties of these solvents were recognized for use in food, aromatherapy, perfume and pharmaceutical industries. Florasol actually comes from the name of the solvent from which it was taken.

Extraction occurs below surrounding temperature level, so there is no occurrence of degradation of the product. The extraction process also uses selective solvents and produces free flowing clear oil, free of waxes.

WHAT CAN AROMATHERAPY HELP WITH?

Aromatherapy is an alternative medicine that primarily uses natural oils as a means of enhancing one's physical and psychological well-being. Many people consider this alternative therapy as a vital part of their daily life since it produces several health benefits. In fact, some of them are now extending the use of aromatherapy to their pets, specifically dogs.

If you have a dog, then you can use aromatherapy for his benefit. It should be noted that aromatherapy typically works through the senses. Aside from the positive effects that your four-legged family member can receive using the sense of touch when you use oils to treat him, he can also gain benefits from the smell and scents.

Remember that a dog's sense of smell is more sensitive than humans, so it is no longer surprising to see aromatherapy getting more and more popular among dog owners. The good thing about dog aromatherapy is that it is versatile that you can use it in treating different problems and conditions affecting your furry friend.

If using it to treat his condition has never come across your mind, then it is time to consider this alternative treatment. However, remember that while it actually offers a host of benefits for him, note that the effects will still depend on the specific oils used in the whole process. Here are some of the safest oils used in dog aromatherapy and how each one can benefit your pet:

- **Cedar Oil** – Using this oil for aromatherapy is a huge help in repelling pests. It works in killing and controlling fleas, ticks, and other parasites. Combined with other inactive ingredients, cedar wood can offer more relaxing and positive effects to dogs. In addition, it also promotes a healthy skin. It can also help calm him, especially during stressful situations.

- **Lavender Oil** – Used in aromatherapy, this oil has several properties that can benefit your pet. What is good about this oil is that you can use it either diluted or pure. One of its benefits to dogs is its sedative and calming action. It is useful in calming fearful, anxious, hyperactive, and agitated dogs. The oil is versatile enough while also having the ability to create a sense of harmony and peace.

  Make it a point to use therapeutic-grade lavender oil for aromatherapy each time your dog faces a stressful situation, such as during a visit to his vet or when you are taking him with you on a trip. It is also useful when you are still training him to quell his hyperactivity. Many dog owners also use lavender oil in aromatherapy for fleas and ticks control. While it does not kill them exactly, it still works in repelling them.

  Lavender also has properties designed to relieve some skin conditions affecting your dog, including dryness and itchiness, thereby promoting better skin health. Aside from all the mentioned benefits, lavender also has a scent which is effective in controlling pet odor.

- **Lemongrass Oil** – One of the many things that lemongrass oil can do when used in dog aromatherapy is to control tick and fleas. Even just a small amount of it is enough to produce a citrus smell that dogs often find pleasant but is actually off-putting when inhaled by ticks and fleas. Such is helpful in driving them away. Aside from that, lemongrass oil also improves your dog's skin condition.

- **Eucalyptus Oil** – Eucalyptus is also a popular and safe oil used in dog aromatherapy. Just like lavender and lemongrass, it is effective in controlling fleas and repelling other parasites. It is also good for your dog's skin as it has soothing effects while offering immediate relief to stings, insect bites, and rashes. It has antiseptic and disinfectant properties, too – all of which are useful in dealing with some skin problems.

  Furthermore, the oil has inhalant properties that work efficiently in combatting respiratory problems, like bronchitis and sinus infections. If you want to control your pet's odor, then the pleasant smell of the oil can help.

- **Frankincense Oil** – If you want to use a less potent and safer essential oil when applying aromatherapy for dog care, then frankincense oil is the answer. The good thing about frankincense is that it is versatile in the sense that you can use it for a number of functions, including wound care, antibacterial healing, and behavior improvement.

- **Clary Sage Oil** – You can also take advantage of the beneficial properties of this oil to dogs. It works in calming their nerves. Another advantage of clary sage oil is that it works gently, provided you only use small amounts of it and dilute it properly. Doing such works in sedating the central nervous system, thereby calming even the most aggressive dogs.

- **Peppermint Oil** – Another essential oil popularly used in aromatherapy is peppermint. It has become popular because of its numerous benefits including its ability to repel parasites and insects and stimulate circulation. It also helps in treating strains, sprains, dysplasia, and arthritis. If you combine the use of the oil with ginger, then you will have an effective solution for motion sickness.

- **Spearmint Oil** – What is good about this essential oil for aromatherapy is that it aids in managing your dog's weight. It is also beneficial in treating nausea, diarrhea, and colic. In addition, it can balance your dog's metabolism, stimulate the proper functioning of his gallbladder, and prevent gastrointestinal issues.

- **Chamomile Oil** – One thing that makes chamomile oil beneficial for dogs is that it has anti-inflammatory properties that are good for their coat and skin. It also lessens allergic reactions. In addition, it is effective in calming nerves and reducing cramps and muscle and teething pain.

- **Cardamom Oil** – It is a natural diuretic, which also contains anti-bacterial properties. It is ideal for dog aromatherapy as it aids in soothing nausea, treating cough, and normalizing his appetite, especially if he tends to eat less than usual.

The oils used in dog aromatherapy contribute a lot on the benefits that your pet can generate. Aside from the already mentioned positive effects, aromatherapy using safe essential oils can also offer the following:

- Offers an invigorating or sedating effect, thereby promoting relaxation to dogs who easily get nervous and anxious
- Calms aggressive behavior and treats hyperactivity and separation anxiety
- Relieves burns, rashes, and other minor skin irritations, including dog allergies
- Relieves joint problems, including growing pains and arthritis
- Prevents and treats gingivitis and bad breath
- Lessens effects of arthritis
- Combats nausea
- Prevents motion and travel sickness
- Reduces the risk of suffering from coughs, respiratory problems, and congestion

The good thing about dog aromatherapy is that its methods are actually easy to implement. In comparison to pills and medicines that offer negative side effects to your dog, aromatherapy is a more natural treatment, making it safe to use. It benefits not only the dog but you, as the pet owner, too.

For instance, giving him a bath using lavender essential oil also gives you the chance to breathe in the oil's aroma. It can then penetrate into your bloodstream through your respiratory system, which is helpful in soothing and relaxing you.

Some Limitations to Take Note of

It should be noted, though, that while aromatherapy offers numerous benefits to dogs, there are still some limitations to it. That said, you need to get the advice of a veterinarian before using the alternative therapy to your dog. Your veterinarian is skilled enough in diagnosing diseases affecting your dog, so you have to consult him/her, especially during those instances when there are severe or persistent symptoms.

Inform your vet about all the natural products that your dog uses and make him/her a part of your decision. Your vet knows exactly what is good and safe for your dog so listen to him. Also, take note that while essential oils help in affecting mentation and healing, they are also very potent, causing plenty of adverse effects if used incorrectly. One main problem in the essential oils used in aromatherapy is that they are rich in adulterants and contaminants that might trigger serious issues.

With that in mind, you really have to be aware of some precautionary and safety measures before implementing this form of alternative therapy to your dog (more about safety measures in the next section of this book). Furthermore, you need to ensure that he is in perfect condition. Make sure that he is not suffering from any health problem that might negatively interact with the oil you are planning to use.

Furthermore, avoid using the therapy for very young or old puppies, as well as for nursing pups and pregnant dogs. Consult your veterinarian first prior to using any treatment, whether it is natural or otherwise.

Overall, dog aromatherapy is one of those forms of treatments designed to help you take good care of your pet. It offers a solid support to the usual traditional veterinary medicine. There are even instances when the therapy replaces the latter. However, you need to be fully aware of how it works. It is also important to gain a full understanding of how certain essential oils affect dogs prior to using them.

The next section of this book will focus more on some precautionary measures that you can apply when using dog aromatherapy just to make sure that your dog stays safe during the whole procedure.

SAFETY MEASURES BEFORE USING ESSENTIAL OILS WITH YOUR DOGS

While essential oils are generally known for being safe and natural, they still have some adverse effects when used incorrectly. If it is your first time to implement dog aromatherapy, then take note that the key to its success is picking the right and safest essential oil and using it correctly. That way, you no longer have to think about the oil causing negative reactions. It should also be noted that in comparison to humans, dogs have a much more acute sense of smell. They have more than 2 million scent receptors present in their nasal passages, making their sense of smell around 10,000-100,000 times more acute than human beings.

They can detect odors in part per trillion. This

means that while it is possible for you to detect that your cup of coffee contains one teaspoon of sugar, your dog can detect one teaspoon of sugar in one million gallons of water. Your dog makes use of his strong sense of smell to generate all forms of information, no matter how complex these are, from their present environment.

They then take advantage of such information to predict and calculate the states of energy and the perfect response for a specific situation. Due to their strong sense of smell, you can expect them to inhale the scent of essential oils rapidly. The scent can then pass via their bloodstream quickly, making aromatherapy one of the most efficient and fast-acting solutions to treating various conditions affecting dogs.

The problem with your dog's strong sense of smell is that it might also cause them to ingest scents and other properties present in certain essential oils that are actually harmful to them. With that in mind, you really have to learn more about essential oils, how to use them safely for dog aromatherapy, and ensure that you are using just enough for his well-being.

The Truth about Essential Oils

Essential oils are actually volatile substances present in glandular hairs, veins, or sacs of various parts of plants, like their bark, flowers, leaves, fruits, roots, and seeds. They are responsible for the unique scents of different plants. Contrary to what a lot of people believe, they are not actually oily. In fact, they are highly concentrated, which is one of the reasons why you need to dilute them prior to each use. Each essential oil also comes with its unique properties, including color, scent, healing effects, and chemical properties.

Since the oils are highly concentrated, they are also extremely potent. That said, you need to be careful when using them to your dogs. Avoid overusing the oils. In addition, it is important to dilute them with a carrier oil, like sweet almond or olive oil, prior to each use. Make sure to look for aromatherapy oils known for their safe effects on dogs, too. They should be in their diluted forms when used so you can safely use them for your dogs and guarantee positive therapeutic effects.

Also, take note that each pet is different, so expect different reactions depending on the essential oil you used and the specific application method you followed. While most of these essential oils are generally safe for dogs, there are certain types that you need to use carefully or avoid completely.

If you are also a cat owner, then you have to be even more cautious when using certain essential oils. It is mainly because cats are sensitive to oils with polyphenolic compounds. Such compounds can negatively interfere with proper liver detoxification.

Assessing the Quality of the Essential Oils

To guarantee the safety of your dog, ensure that you invest in high-quality essential oils. Note that there are low-quality ones out there that contain lots of harmful and toxic chemicals and substances. Check whether the essential oils you are planning to buy are of top-notch quality with the aid of these guidelines:

- **Be wary of low-priced oils** – Do not go for essential oils offered at extremely low prices as there is a chance that they are low in quality. Go for a reasonably priced brand, which already established a good reputation in the industry. Also, take note that most high-quality essential oils are expensive, so avoid unreasonably low-priced ones as there is a chance that they are also adulterated.

Avoid buying the oils at health food stores or supermarkets, too. While they are cheaper, most of them are of low quality.

- **Choose organic oil** – Buying an organic variety is crucial in preventing the risk of pesticide contamination. The majority of brands actually carry the official seal of USDA, but it is important to find an oil, which has the word "wild-crafted" on its label. This means that the oil was created using a plant harvested in the wild. The plant is not farmed, meaning it does not contain chemicals sprayed by farmers.

- **Check if the label indicates that it is 100% pure** – If it does not have such phrase in the label, then there is a great chance that it is altered. There is also a chance that another ingredient is used in it. If you want to use an essential oil, which can really improve the health and well-being of your dog, then make sure that it is pure and does not contain any unwanted and unnecessary chemicals and substances. Another sign that you are getting a high-quality and pure essential oil is if it is in cobalt, violet, or amber glass bottles.

- **Look for vital information about the oils** – You can find the information on the label, in the brochure, or the store's official website. Some of the information you have to find are its Latin name, common name, method of extraction, country of origin and cultivation method – ex. cultivated, organic, and wild-harvested. There should also be 100% pure essential oil printed on its label.

If you have a hard time finding such details from the store's provided resources, including its label, then consider this as a red flag. The provider of the product should make it easy for you to obtain some important information about the oils.

Some Safety and Precautionary Measures

Aside from learning about the essential oils that you should avoid as well as how to assess their quality, you also have to take note of some safety and precautionary measures when using them for dog aromatherapy.

1. *Use high-quality, therapeutic-grade oils* – These are the safest oils that you can use for dogs. Low quality ones often contain additives while being stretched by adding multiple carrier oils, leading to pet sensitivities. There are also low quality ones made by combining oils with other absolutes or botanicals resembling certain scents. They are actually unhealthy not only for your dog but also for you because they contain solvents.

   That said, make sure to choose pure and therapeutic brands of essential oils offered by reputable companies. Use the guidelines mentioned earlier to assess their quality. Ensure that they do not contain any added chemicals, too. If you want your dog to ingest the oils directly, the labels should indicate that they are indeed "for internal use". If you can avoid it, though, do not let your dog ingest the oils directly as doing so might harm him. Check the labels, too, to determine if there are clear instructions in diluting the oils, ensuring their proper and safe use.

2. *Dilute the essential oils* – Excess use of the oils might lead to liver failure and

might also trigger skin irritation. If you use undiluted ones, then there is a tendency for your pet's sensitive sense of smell to be affected. Dogs' sense of smell are more sensitive when compared to humans, so diluting the oils even if you just want your pet to inhale them is important in addressing common concerns related to safety.

To dilute, a rough guide is to mix around 3-6 drops of your chosen essential oils to 30-ml or 1-ounce carrier oil. Some of the carrier oils that are safe for this purpose are olive, sweet almond and jojoba oil. If you are still a beginner in using aromatherapy oils, then consider doing a patch test first to check for allergies or sensitivities.

Do this by applying a small drop of the oil you are planning to use on a concealed area. A good place is the skin found on the upper inner part of his leg. Leave it for 24 hours then check again to find out of there is any irritation, redness or swelling.

3. *Use a high-quality aromatherapy diffuser* – As has been mentioned earlier, dogs have a strong sense of

smell, so the common mistake committed by pet owners is using the oil excessively. To avoid such mistake, make it a point to use a high-quality aromatherapy diffuser. With the help of this diffuser, you will have full control over the amount of emitted oil. Look for a high-quality diffuser as it can help diffuse just the right amount into the air, thereby preventing you and your dog from getting too overwhelmed with the scent and its effects.

4. *Test the oil's purity* – Before using the essential oil, you need to have a guarantee that it is 100% pure. Even if the label indicates that it is pure, you have to be sure by testing its purity right after you purchase it. You can do this test by putting one drop of the oil into a piece of paper. Let it dry. You will instantly know that the oil is not pure if it leaves behind an oil ring into the white paper.

Note, though, that there are certain exceptions to this rule. It is because there are certain oils that are heavier in terms of consistency and deeper in color – ex. German chamomile, patchouli oils, and sandalwood. Such might still leave some tint behind. In this case, your goal should be to check if the tint is greasy as the grease signifies that it is not pure.

5. *Use the aromatherapy oils only to address a concern affecting your dog and not as a means of preventing a specific health condition* – For instance, avoid letting your dog inhale the oil after eating even if you know that he does not have a digestive problem. Dog aromatherapy is not meant to treat a problem which is not yet there.

6. *Consult your veterinarian* – Before using any oil, ask your vet about it first. Find out if it is really safe to use for your dog. You need a vet's advice especially if he is below ten weeks old, pregnant, or has an existing medical condition. It is also important to consult him regarding the proper use of the oil based on the breed, size, health history, and age.

7. *Consider the size of your dog* – If he is small, then he is more prone to experiencing the usual harmful side effects of the oil, so consider using or applying only a small amount. When diluting, take into consideration his actual size. Also, avoid using the oils on

puppies below eight weeks old who come from medium to large breed. If you have a small breed puppy, however, then you can safely use the oils but make sure that he is already at least ten weeks. That's the safest time for you to apply the oils.

8. *Introduce the oils in a positive environment* – What you can do is to let him smell it first then wait for a while to check for signs of acceptance. Some signs that will let you know that your dog accepts the oils are when he rubs himself against you and when he wants to lick the oil. If there is a positive response, then you can apply the oil. However, if you notice that he turns his head away or do some other things, like whining, sneezing, pacing, drooling, or panting, then it signifies that he does not like the oil, so you need to use a different one.

9. *Do not use the essential oils on sensitive areas* – Some of the areas where you should avoid applying the diluted oil into are the genitals, anal area, eyes and nose. You actually have no reason to put it on the mentioned areas, so avoid doing so as much as possible if you do

not want your dog to feel extremely uncomfortable.

Probably the most important among the tips already mentioned is to avoid adding the essential oil to your dog's drinking water or food. Any form of direct ingestion should be avoided as it is not meant for that purpose. Use the other aromatherapy applications that we will discuss later instead of direct ingestion.

IS AROMATHERAPY SUITABLE FOR YOUR DOG?

Just like how useful aromatherapy is for humans, it is also beneficial for pets, especially dogs who need healing because of its therapeutic and positive emotional effects. With the therapy's increasing number of benefits, it is no longer surprising to see it as a popular alternative healing technique designed to cure a variety of health-related and emotional issues affecting dogs. It is designed to deal with emotional disorders and physical diseases.

If your dog lives indoors, then he might have already lost his primal abilities. In most cases, dogs who freely roam outdoors look happier because they have the opportunity to run around and do what they want the entire day

However, they also spend their day smelling almost all kinds of things, particularly those that are in their purest and most natural form. Letting them sniff and smell the beneficial aromatherapy oils is a big help in healing any physical and emotional disorders that they have.

The question now is whether or not aromatherapy oils are really suitable for your dog. You don't want to put his health condition at risk, do you? So there is a chance that you would want to conduct an extensive research first prior to exposing him to any essential oil. Note that while aromatherapy makes use of essential oils designed to produce scents enjoyed by humans, there are also volatile substances and compounds present in the oils, making them potentially toxic when used to your dog at specific concentrations.

Also, take note that dogs are sensitive to these essential oils. With that in mind, you will realize that what is actually safe for people does not necessarily mean that it is safe for your dog, too. Not applying it correctly and on the right place might cause your dog to inhale, eat, or lick the oils inadvertently. There is also a chance for his skin to absorb the oils.

Since dogs react differently when exposed to these substances, it is essential to discuss your plan to use aromatherapy oils with your vet and listen to what he has to say about it. Make sure that your furry friend won't really experience pain, discomfort, or other health issues due to it.

Are Aromatherapy Oils Safe for your Dog?

Generally, all dog breeds can safely use aromatherapy oils. However, you have to take extreme caution especially if he is from a breed that is prone to or has existing breathing problems. Some dog breeds that commonly suffer from breathing problems, like brachycephalic airway syndrome, are pug, boxer, bulldog, Shih Tzu, Staffordshire bull terrier, Boston terrier, and Pekingese. If your dog is from any of the mentioned breeds, then be extra cautious in implementing any of the aromatherapy methods.

Talk to your vet first and ask for a professional opinion to determine if it is safe to use aromatherapy and the corresponding essential oils even if your pet is prone to breathing problems or difficulties. Also, keep in mind that while the majority of dogs have less or zero problems when it comes to using essential oils, you need to be extra careful if you are still new to using this alternative therapy to dogs.

As a rule of thumb, puppies who are from medium to large breeds, like the German shepherd, Labrador retriever, Otter hound, and Saint Bernard, who are not yet 10 weeks of age should never be exposed to aromatherapy oils. It is because the substances are not yet safe for puppies of the mentioned breeds who are around that age. Wait for them to reach ten weeks before starting to implement aromatherapy.

Another rule to keep in mind is to avoid using the oils on toy dogs, as well as pregnant and old ones. It is mainly because these are among the most sensitive types of pets, requiring additional care. You can't expose them to certain elements and substances that may only have a negative impact on their overall health. Aromatherapy oil is not suitable for epileptic dogs, too.

How to Determine if an Essential Oil is Safe for your Dog?

Animals, especially dogs, metabolize and react in a much different way to essential oils than humans, so it is crucial to know about such differences to avoid any negative reactions. One common problem encountered is overusing the oils. There are instances when dog owners diffuse too much oils into their households, causing unintentional overdose for dogs. You can avoid this from happening by testing your dog's reaction to the oil first and figuring out the safest dose for him.

Fortunately, there are a few tests designed to help you determine the suitability and safety of an essential oil for dogs. For instance, if your dog has never smelled any natural or essential oil in the past, then let him sniff your chosen mixture first and observe his initial reaction. If he responds negatively, then it may not be the best and safest oil for him. However, it is still possible for you to make him get used to the smell.

What you have to do is to place the aromatherapy oil in a diluted mist form. Spray a bit of it in the place where he sleeps and usually roam around. That way, he can start getting used to the smell. If you can't still get him to like the oil, then maybe it is not really suitable for him so it is advisable to look for another one, which he can easily adopt.

If your pet is sensitive, then make sure to check

for any signs of negative reaction. Use small doses first. Avoid using your chosen oil at full strength if it is still the first time for your dog to get exposed to it.

Another tip is to pre-select around three to five essential oils from the ones known to be safe for them. Make sure that your choice also depends on the specific issue that you want to address. Pre-selecting at least three beneficial oils will let you choose one, which your dog particularly likes and is suitable for his specific condition and needs.

Once you have made the selection, offer each oil to him one at a time. Each one should still be in a closed bottle when you offer it to your dog. Let him sniff the bottle while it is closed. Keep in mind that with your dog's excellent sense of smell, he can sniff the scent even if it is closed.

Observe his reaction so you will know which one he really likes. Some of the signs and reactions to watch out for that might indicate that the oil does not suit your dog are nervousness, whining, and excessive scratching. Once you determined the oil preferred by your dog, dilute it accordingly. You can then start offering it to him again through inhalation.

Also, ensure that you use oils that are safe and suitable for most dogs. Keep in mind that there are those that are not suitable for them, posing dangers especially when used in extremely large amounts. Avoid using the following essential oils, too, as they are not safe for dogs and might only trigger skin sensitivities, allergies, and interference to their natural body functions.

- **Camphor, White Thyme, Juniper, Yarrow and Anise** – All these oils can trigger possible toxicity or uterine stimulation, so avoid using them on your dog, especially if pregnant ones. As for juniper, you can actually use the juniper berry oil variety as it is safe for dogs. However, do not use juniper wood oil as it is toxic to the kidneys.

- **Wintergreen and Birch** – While you can actually use these aromatherapy oils for joint pains and arthritis, it is not ideal for dermal or skin purposes. It is because of their toxic properties caused by the high methyl salicylate content. Ensure that your dog does not ingest it in any way, too, as it might lead to severe poisoning, and even death.

- **Clove Leaf and Bud** – Avoid these oils, too, because these tend to trigger dermal irritation. They can also lead to toxicity not only to your dog but also to you and the people around.

- **Horseradish and Mustard** – Both of these oils have pungent properties, making them risky when used on dogs. They may also trigger severe dermal irritation.

- **Wormwood** – Wormwood is toxic to pets, particularly dogs, so make sure to avoid it as much as possible. It triggers seizures while also holding high dermal and oral toxicity.

- **Oregano** – It is a toxic oil for dogs so avoid using it as much as possible. However, there are still instances when you can use it but only in extremely small amounts and after you diluted it properly with a carrier oil. Such results to an aromatherapy solution, which is good for dogs who have poor respiratory health. Despite that, it is important for you to spend time weighing all the risks involved in applying the oregano oil. Also, consider vital factors, like your dog's breed, size, and age, and discuss this with your vet first.

- **Tea Tree** – Tea tree oil can also put your dog at risk, especially if you use extremely high doses. It is still beneficial but only in small amounts. Ensure that your dog does not have too much contact with tea tree.

Make it a point to use other essential oils in dog aromatherapy, instead of the ones mentioned above, to guarantee his safety. Note that while aromatherapy for dogs is extremely beneficial for his overall health, there are also risks if you choose to apply one, which is not suitable for him.

Typical Safety Precautions When Using Essential Oils on Canines

- Use essential oils that are safe and 100 percent pure on dogs and humans.
- Be sure to dilute essential oils before using on dogs. For a rough guide, add 5-6 drops of essential oil to 1 ounce or 30 ml. of carrier base oil. For 8 ounces or 240 ml. of shampoo, use 20-25 drops of essential oils.
- Use smaller amounts of diluted oil on smaller dogs, puppies and aged dogs whose health is compromised. If you are not sure if your dog's current condition can take essential oils, then start off with hydrosols.
- Never use essential oils on dogs with epilepsy or who are prone to seizure attacks. Some oils such as rosemary can trigger seizures even in humans.
- Avoid applying essential oils around the eyes, or close to the nose, anal or genital organs. These areas contain easily irritated membranes and can be susceptible to increased chemical absorption.

- Do not fail to check with a holistic veterinarian before using any essential oils on pregnant dogs. Essential oils like peppermint, eucalyptus, tea tree and rosemary must be avoided especially when your dog is pregnant.
- Some oils are not suitable for use on dogs ever, in any quantity. Phenols, such as those in Oregano and Thyme oils are not indicated for use on canines. Pennyroyal and Wormwood oils should never be used. Be sure to only use recipes that you trust, from sources that are educated in aromatherapy and holistic veterinarian practice.
- If your animal has a history of sensitive skin, be sure to patch test any topical treatment on a small area of skin before applying fully. The skin is a complicated organ and it can be hard to predict its reaction. A patch test is the safest way to prevent a large and possibly painful amount of irritation.

- Some oils can increase sensitivity to sunlight. Citrus oils, in particular, are known for this. On short-haired breeds especially, it is very important to make sure your dog's skin is not exposed to these oils and sunlight at the same time. Doing so can increase the risk of sunburn, possibly to a large degree. Ears are a particular area of concern, because in many breeds they tend to be sunlight sensitive to begin with.
- Never assume that an oil that is safe in one application is safe in another. Some oils are therapeutic when applied topically but useless or, even worse, toxic if taken internally. This is why it is important to follow recipe and application instructions very carefully. Not only that, but make sure the source of your recipe is a trusted and educated source.
- Always make sure your supply of essential oils, carrier oils and mixtures made with them are stored properly. Above all: they must be stored out of the reach of

your animals. Some oils can smell quite tasty to dogs, but if they are ingested in any but the smallest quantities they are toxic. Even a neutral oil like vegetable oil will cause digestive troubles if eaten in large amounts. Treat these ingredients and remedies as you would any other medicine by making sure there is no way your dog can access them. If you ever suspect that your dog has obtained access to them, monitor them very closely for symptoms and call your veterinarian.

- Tea Tree oil is a common home remedy for bacterial issues. However, it can be too strong for dogs, especially small ones. If you do decide to use it, be cautious at first, always do a patch test and limit the duration of exposure. Also consider that you may be able to swap Sweet Marjoram oil for it and still achieve the desired effect.
- "Hot spots" like at the joint of the legs or neck may be more sensitive to topical applications than the spine or sides would

be. On animals with a lot of fur or skin, keep in mind that where the skin meets skin or stays much warmer, it can intensify the effect of the oil. If it is necessary to apply remedies to these areas, keep in mind that it may be advisable to dilute the mixture to account for this. A patch test is helpful in this instance as well.

- When using a diffuser to disperse essential oils in your home there are a few precautions that will make it safer. First, turn diffusers off when you aren't at home. Dogs are more sensitive to smells than we are, so without being able to see and monitor your pet, there is no way to know if the scent has become too strong. Secondly, keep your diffuser clean. If it becomes contaminated with dust, mold or other particulate matter, those will be diffused through your home as well. This can cause all sorts of irritation and problems and is very easy to avoid.
- Consider carrier oils carefully. Depending

on your dog's skin and where the mixture is being applied, you may see a range of reactions. With a patch test, for instance, you may see dryness or slight irritation. Sometimes this is not due to the essential oil at all, but to the carrier oil. Oils like Avocado or Coconut may simply be too heavy for your animal's particular skin and fur needs. Conversely, mildly astringent oils like Mint or Rosemary may cause irritation when blended with a very lightweight oil like Apricot Seed, but could be perfect when carried in something richer. If skin sensitivity is a concern, patch test all carrier oils on their own so you can see how your dog reacts before mixing other essential oils in.

DIFFERENT AROMATHERPY APPLICATIONS

Due to the many benefits of essential oils, it is safe to say that these serve as powerful tools in the health care toolkit of your dogs. Using them properly and correctly in aromatherapy can help you deal with the most common concerns affecting dogs, including anxiety and stress. The good thing about aromatherapy oils is that they are natural. This means that you can improve the health condition of your dog without sedation or intense drugs. All that you need is the natural soothing power provided by the aromatherapy oils.

Even small amounts of the oils can already help in treating a host of health conditions and problems. It heals the entire body – both physically and emotionally. In addition, the oils contain plenty of antiseptic, revitalizing, detoxifying, regulating, anti-microbial, and calming properties, making them truly valuable for both humans and dogs.

However, it is important to understand how to use and apply it properly. Used correctly, the oils serve as gentle, safe, and natural solutions for treating various dog problems without any side effects. Aromatherapy serves as a great solution for allergies, fear, anxiety, liver function, joint problems, skin conditions, and other issues that hamper the overall health condition of your dog.

The Different Application Methods

You have a few options when it comes to applying the aromatherapy oils into your dog. Just make sure that whichever method you choose, you prioritize his safety. Here are some of the ways for you to apply the oils on your dog safely and ensure that he will get all the benefits promised by aromatherapy.

1. **Massage** – Prior to massaging your chosen oil into his skin, dilute it first. Dilute it in a base oil before massaging on the affected area. Once in the diluted form, you can gently massage it into a hairless part of your dog's skin, like the

inner thigh, groin, or armpit. You can also go to the part with the least amount of hair. Do this for around three to four minutes.

If you choose to apply the aromatherapy oils directly into his skin through a gentle massage, then a wise tip is to only cover those areas starting from his neck to his tail. Choose oils that can quickly penetrate into his skin, too, so he can start enjoying the effects as soon as possible. However, you need to avoid applying the oil directly or close to his face, nose, or eyes. Prevent it from getting ingested internally, too.

In this case, be careful when massaging the oil. Make it a point to put the oil in a part of his body where he can't lick. However, even if the massage application only involves applying the oil externally, you should still avoid doing it if your dog is pregnant or prone to seizures. Only do it once you receive the go-signal of your vet.

2. **Diffuser** – You can also try aromatherapy for dogs using a diffuser. In this case, you need to combine your chosen aromatherapy oil with a source

of heat. The good news is that you have plenty of options when it comes to using a diffuser for dog aromatherapy.

For instance, you can go for those diffusers that operate using electricity. There are also those that require candles. Another option is a ring-shaped device, which you need to place on the topmost part of a light bulb. To use your chosen diffuser, follow these guidelines:

- Place the recommended number of drops of your chosen essential oil into the diffuser. Doing this will prompt the scents of the aromatherapy oil to instantly fill up the room.

- Let your dog stay in the room filled up with the scent for around thirty minutes. This will allow him to breathe in the oil as it evaporates into the air.

- To guarantee better results, consider doing this two times daily. Done properly, it is possible for you to see positive results within 5-7 days.

If you decide to use a diffuser, though, ensure that your dog has an escape route just in case he does not like the scent produced by the oil. With an escape route, he can easily get out of the room right away if he starts to feel uncomfortable.

3. **Topical application** – This is a popular way to use aromatherapy for dogs. In this form of application, you will need to apply your chosen oil directly into the needed area/s. Such will let the oil penetrate deeply into the skin. The small capillaries will then absorb it quickly, carrying the oils into the bloodstream. You can actually apply your chosen aromatherapy oil to your dog topically via massage, which has already been explained earlier.

Another way to apply it topically is with the help of sprays or spritzers. You also have the option to put it on dog shampoo, conditioner, ointment, or salve and apply it to your pet topically using the mentioned products. Diluting the oil should be the first thing you have to do before using it topically. In this case, you can make use of carrier oils, including sweet almond, jojoba, or olive oil.

4. **Petting** – If you want a less intense topical application of aromatherapy oil to your dog, then petting is an ideal option. What you have to do is to place the diluted oil into your hands. Rub your hands containing the oil until it produces a light film based on your preferred concentration.

   Use both your hands to pet the dog with the oil. This is a less intense technique of using aromatherapy to address common emotional issues affecting dogs, like depression, stress, and anxiety. Petting and the diluted oil both work in calming him down.

Regardless of which method you choose, make sure to use a high-quality essential oil for it. Also, remember not to be tempted to put the oil into his food nor rub it on him even if you noticed that he does not want it. Avoid forcing the oil on him as doing so might cause adverse reactions. Use only those aromatherapy oils that draw a positive response from him.

Basic Rules Before the Final Application

To ensure that you apply the aromatherapy oils correctly using any of the approaches mentioned above, you have to be fully aware of the basic rules involved in it. One is to decide on the specific oil that should help your dog first. What you have to do is to create a shortlist of at least five aromatherapy oils. Put each one in a closed bottle then let each settle on your floor with enough spaces in between.

Encourage your dog to come close to the bottles and smell them. Observe and figure out which one among the closed bottles he sniffs intently or in some cases, tries to lick. Your dog will most likely stop sniffing once he finally reached the oil he wants and needs. Let him make the choice as he actually has the ability to pick exactly the one he needs. Note that each dog has the ability to pick the exact oil required for his condition, so give him a chance to guide his own healing through this activity.

Make sure that you fully understand a dog's major responses to the oils, too. In most cases, dogs use three major ways to respond to the aromatic extracts. These are smelling/inhalation, localized topical application, and licking. Inhalation is considered to be the most powerful because the oils tend to go directly to the brain using the dog's olfactory system, which then alters his brain chemistry.

In most cases, your dog will also show you what he wants you to do with the oil by pointing his head into a specific part of his body, moving into you, or stamping his foot. If he does any of these, then note that he might want you to apply the oil on a specific part of his body topically, usually in an acupuncture point. When this happens, just rub a small amount of the oil into the indicated body part.

Diluting the Oil

After choosing a specific oil, diluting it should follow. This is an important step you should not neglect as the undiluted form may be too strong and powerful for your dog to handle. If you use too much of the oil in its undiluted form, then your dog might deal with adverse reactions, such as skin irritation and liver failure. You can dilute it by mixing around 1-3 drops of the oil in a teaspoon of cold-pressed vegetable oil – ex. olive or sunflower oil. Once diluted, you can offer it to your dog then observe how he responds to it.

If there is a positive response, then you can start offering this to him based on your chosen application one to two times daily. Do this routine until he starts losing interest in the oil. There is a chance for him to lose interest in the diluted oil within 3 days to one week. If this happens, you will also notice a significant change in the problem you are planning to treat.

If you have young pups, old dogs, or those who are sick causing them to require special care and attention, then avoid giving them too much of the oil. Note that increasing the dosage won't be of help at all in the mentioned cases. In fact, if you are still in doubt, a wise advice is to use lesser amount of the diluted oil than what is recommended. You can also utilize a diffuser initially just to be safe.

Despite being in their diluted form, you have to take note that the essential oils are strong, so you should avoid direct contact to your dog's eye area, inner ear, or face. If you plan to use it on his tummy, then focus on what you are doing to avoid the risk of the oil reaching his anal or genital area.

Consider your Dog Breed's Size

Before the final application, keep in mind that the size of your dog contributes a lot on the specific amount of essential oil you need to use. If you have a small dog breed, then three to five drops are already more than enough. Dilute around 80 to 90% of it before application. If you have large dogs, then begin with three to five drops. In this case, you can use the undiluted oils unless the product label instructs you to do otherwise.

For giant dog breeds, like a Great Dane, you can still give them diluted essential oils but consider increasing the dosage - at least 6 drops will do. For very small pups, such as a tiny Yorkie, around 1-2 drops are often enough. You need to avoid overdosing your dog with the oil, so be extra cautious when applying the products.

AROMATHERAPY TOOLS AND MATERIALS

For you to start taking full advantage of aromatherapy for dogs, you need to gather a few tools and materials. This chapter will talk about everything that you will most likely need once you decide to introduce aromatherapy oils to your dog. If you have all these tools and materials, then making the most out of the oils in terms of improving your dog's health is possible.

Essential Oils

Of course, you need a collection of essential oils known to be safe for dogs. You can refer to a previous chapter of this book to determine which oils are safe to use for pets, especially dogs, and which ones are not. Before making your choice out of the many essential oils today, have a vet check your dog first to figure out if the one you intend to use is safe for him.

Such is crucial in determining if he has an undiagnosed health problem that might negatively react to the procedure. Also, if you want to make a more modest investment with essential oils, consider purchasing those in 5-ml bottles first. Take note of some of the most expensive varieties, like the Frankincense and chamomile, and determine if you are willing to shell out more money for them.

Carrier Oils

Carrier oils are also among the most important items you need before you can start taking advantage of aromatherapy for dogs. In fact, they serve as the foundation of the majority of blends. You can use them in diluting the essential oils so they will be safe to apply on your dog's skin.

With a good collection of safe carrier oils, you can produce diluted forms of the essential oils that you can safely distribute to the different parts of your dog's body. Some of the best carrier oils that are suitable for dog aromatherapy are olive, coconut, sunflower, apricot, grape seed, and sweet almond oil.

Measuring Spoons and Cups

Once you decide to make your own aromatherapy blends for dogs, it is necessary for you to invest in a separate set of measuring spoons and cups from the ones in your kitchen. Make sure to use these items only for the purpose of measuring ingredients for the blends. As mentioned in some parts of this book, dogs are sensitive. They have a strong sense of smell.

With that in mind, you have to make sure that your blends have the right amount of essential and carrier oils, as well as other ingredients. Inaccurate measurement might lead to producing aromatherapy blends that might harm your dog, instead of healing him.

If you plan to measure large quantities, then it would be best to have a Pyrex measuring cup, which also comes with a pour spout. Your measuring spoon also plays a major role as you can use it to measure essential oils accurately, especially if you need more than just a few drops.

Bottles/Containers

Bottles and other containers should also form part of the tools you own for aromatherapy. A few bottles, jars, and other containers are crucial if you want to store your produced blend properly. Some bottles and containers that you can use for the safe storage of the blends are the following:

- *Amber Glass Bottle* – Consider getting one with a secure lid. You can also go for amber glass bottles with droppers as these promote ease in adding the correct number of drops needed for a specific situation. Make sure to go for nice bottles that are dark enough to ensure that the blends inside are protected while still allowing you to see exactly what is inside and how much is already left.

- *Glass Roller Bottle* – A glass roller bottle is also another of those supplies that you will love to have on hand for use in dog aromatherapy. You can go for small 10-ml bottles that have roller ball tops in producing your own blends. With the roller top, you can easily apply the aromatherapy blends to your dog then store the bottle somewhere safe once you are done using it.

- *Glass Spray Bottle* – You can also make use of this specific container if you plan to take advantage of aromatherapy for dogs through inhalation. You just need to put your created blends in this bottle then spray some in a room where your dog often stays.

No matter what type of bottles or containers you use for storing your produced aromatherapy blends, ensure that they are securely covered. Also, make sure that they are made of materials and come in colors that will let you clearly see what is inside. It is also advisable to label each container. Put the exact date you made it, the ingredients, name of the blend, or any other important details in the label. That way, you won't end up using the wrong one for your dog.

Diffuser

It is also essential for you to invest in a good quality diffuser. Note that diffusing essential oils into the air, especially if your dog is in an enclosed space, such as a room in your house or his kennel, is one of the most effective applications of aromatherapy for dogs. Such allows the sweet-smelling and highly aromatic molecules of essential oils to be breathed in by the dogs, stimulating several healing, stimulation, relaxation, and immune-boosting responses.

The good thing about having a high-quality diffuser is that it lets you diffuse oil into the kennel or your home, which aids in naturally purifying air by getting rid of toxins, harmful microscopic debris, and metallic particles. It also inhibits the reproduction and growth of airborne pathogens, letting you and your pet stay in a safe and healthy environment. The following are just some of the types of diffusers that are suitable for dog aromatherapy:

- *Cold Air Diffuser* – This type of diffuser utilizes room temperature air as a means of blowing your chosen oil into the nebulizer. The goal is to vaporize the oil into the air. What makes this type of diffuser useful is that it works quickly and efficiently. However, it is not that effective in diffusing thicker and heavier essential oils. Many also find it a bit difficult to clean.

- *Evaporative Diffuser* – Another choice is the evaporative diffuser. It has a basic operation, which involves the use of a fan as a means of blowing air through a filter or pad where you put the oil. Such works in vaporizing the oil that you placed in the pad. This diffuser also covers glass pendants, inhalers, and clay pendants.

There is a drawback, though, such as the fact that it tends to diffuse lighter oils, like citrus, faster than heavier ones. It is more suitable for use when you and your dog are inside your vehicle or during those times when you bring him on a trip.

- *Heat Diffuser* – This is the perfect choice for you if you want to spread a pleasant smell around your home. It aids in producing a nice smell that can soothe or relax your dog. However, if you want to take full advantage of the therapeutic and healing properties present in essential oils, then it would be best to stay away from heat diffuser.

  It is because heat has the tendency of changing the oil's properties and chemistries. It can then result to removing the therapeutic and healing properties it has. It would be best to use this diffuser if your goal is just to make your entire home or the specific area your dog is staying in smell more pleasantly.

- *Ultrasonic Diffuser* – This is the best choice especially if you want to make the most out of all the therapeutic benefits and healing properties present in your chosen oil. This diffuser utilizes electronic frequencies as a means of creating vibrations in water. Such vibrations will then be brought into the surface where there are floating essential oils.

With the help of the vibrations, the oils will be vaporized, dispersing their scents and properties into the air – that is possible even if you do not use a source of heat. In comparison to heat diffuser, it does not damage the healing properties of the oils you decide to use. It works efficiently in purifying air while also getting rid of any unwanted odor.

Choose one diffuser, which you think is really effective in spreading the therapeutic benefits of the oil and letting your dog enjoy them.

Storage Box or Shelf

Of course, you also need to invest in a storage box or shelf where you can safely store or place your aromatherapy blends for dogs. You can't mix it with all the other stuff present in your home. You need a separate storage place where you can keep them all together so you won't end up mixing things up and using the wrong stuff for your dog.

The best storage box or shelf is one which allows you to store not only your aromatherapy blends but also all the tools and supplies that you need for the procedure.

Aside from the mentioned tools and supplies, it is also advisable to have a good reference guide or book. This is important especially if you are still a beginner in using aromatherapy for dogs. Even if you are still a beginner, you will feel more at ease with the right reference guide around as you know that you are well-guided in terms of proper use, how to blend certain ingredients, dilution ratios, and other important stuff.

3 GREAT AROMATHERAPIES FOR YOUR DOG

In the last section of this book, you will get to know about three of the best aromatherapy recipes that you can use for your dog and some bonus recipes/blends. The good thing about the recipes here is that they are designed in such a way that they can treat or deal with a number of conditions affecting your dog.

For Easily Stressed, Anxious, and Fearful Dogs

If you have a dog who tends to get easily stressed and anxious, then the aromatherapy blend below will definitely help him. Note that just like humans, dogs are also prone to experiencing some negative emotions, like separation anxiety, fear, nervousness, and stress.

The good news is that you can now address the mentioned issues with the help of therapeutic-grade essential oils. The following recipe is designed to calm and soothe dogs, ensuring that he does not get too stressed out, anxious or fearful in certain situations.

Ingredients:

- 300-ml water
- 5 to 10 drops Roman chamomile essential oil
- 5 to 10 drops lavender essential oil

Instructions:

1. Combine all the ingredients in a bowl. Pour the mixture in a spray bottle. Shake it to mix everything well.

2. Cover the eyes and face of your dog. You can use your hand or a clean cloth as cover and prevent the oil from penetrating the mentioned areas.

3. Spray a light mist around your dog in those instances when he gets anxious, stressed out, or nervous. It can help settle him down. Another option is spraying a mist into your palms then

applying the blend through massage. Massage his back, chest, and neck as it can calm him down.

Another variation of the recipe is to use 5 drops each of cedar wood and lavender and mix them in the same amount of water mentioned earlier before putting the blend in a spray bottle. Follow the same instructions above when applying it to your dog. You can also use a diffuser but you have to reduce the amount of essential oils needed.

You can just use one drop of cedar wood, lavender or the chamomile, put enough water in the diffuser then pour the oil into it. Turn the diffuser on to calm your anxious, nervous or fearful dog. Expect the result of this recipe and its variations to offer soothing effects in as little as thirty minutes.

The best time to take advantage of this aromatherapy blend for dogs is ten minutes before you leave home or before the arrival of your guests.

For Flea & Tick Removal

One of the most common issues affecting dogs that aromatherapy oils can treat is the presence of fleas and ticks. Fortunately, it is not that hard to create a recipe designed to remove fleas and ticks and ensure that your dog will no longer deal with the side effects of having them around. Here is one simple recipe that you can try to finally get rid of the problem.

Ingredients:

- 1 drop cedar wood
- 5 drops lavender
- 2 drops citronella
- 1 cup water – Consider doubling this amount if you have a dog who is too sensitive to smell.

Instructions:

1. Get a bowl and mix all the mentioned ingredients well with the aid of a wire whisk.

2. Soak cotton bandannas into it. Allow the bandannas to dry naturally in the sun. You can also use it for dog collars. Just make sure to avoid letting the blend get into the plastic parts of the collars. Note that some essential oils tend to degrade the plastic so be careful.

3. After drying the bandana or dog collar, put it around his neck. In case he is too sensitive to smell, then consider tying

the bandana or collar to his harness before taking him for walks. Put it in a place away from his nose.

You can also create a spray version of this recipe, which can repel ticks and fleas naturally. You just need 5 drops of lavender, 2 tablespoons carrier oil and 2 drops each of citronella, lemongrass, and cedar wood. A 10 to 12-ounce spray bottle is also essential in storing the blend after mixing them. Go for a bottle with a 16-ounce capacity, though, especially if you noticed that the blend has a strong scent.

Spray it around your dog while avoiding all parts of his face, including the eyes. You can also spray it just around your house. Because your dog has a strong sense of smell, he can definitely pick up the scent of the aromatherapy blend and enjoy its benefits. If you decide to add more oils than what have been mentioned, then consider reducing the number of drops you use, too. Such is crucial in preventing the final scent from becoming too overwhelming for your dog to handle.

For Proper Skin Health and Support

Your dog's skin can also greatly benefit from certain aromatherapy recipes and blends. If your dog is prone to itchiness, dryness, and other skin irritations, then you can make use of essential oils designed to get rid of the problem and promote better skin health. Aromatherapy oils also help in supporting an aging dog's skin, thereby keeping it healthy no matter how old he is. One recipe designed to promote better skin health in dogs is the following:

Ingredients:

- 5 drops lavender
- 2 tablespoons carrier oil – Your options include olive or jojoba oil.
- 3 drops each of frankincense and Roman chamomile
- 3 drops Vitamin E

Instructions:

1. Combine all the mentioned ingredients in a bowl or measuring cup. Once done, pour the mixture into a roller ball bottle or a dropper bottle. Go for glass-based bottles so you can easily check and monitor the content.

2. Put on two to four drops of the blend to your dog's skin. It is a huge help in maintaining the excellent health of the skin of aging dogs. You can also use it

for skin patches that are dry as the blend works in adding moisture to the area.

Aside from the three recipes already mentioned, it is also possible for you to create the following at home with the aid of aromatherapy oils – all of these are designed to improve the overall health and well-being of your dog:

1. **Deodorizing Spray** – Consider making this spray at home, especially if your dog often goes outdoors for long hours and comes back home with an unwanted smell. The only things that you need for this are 5-ounce water, 5 drops lavender essential oil, 15 drops purification oil, and a pinch of salt. Mix the oils with the salt first then stir it gently before pouring the mixture to the water. Spray this blend to your dog to guarantee instant odor relief.

2. **Immune-strengthening Spray** – This easy-to-make spray is designed to strengthen the immune system of your dog. All you need are 5 drops each of lavender and frankincense and just enough water to fill up a 12-ounce spray bottle. Just mix the oils then pour it into

the bottle filled with water. Seal it with the lid. Spray it on your dog, avoiding any part of his face as much as possible. You can also massage it on certain parts, like his chest, back, and neck.

3. **Muscle Ache Relief** – If you have an active dog, then there is a great chance for him to overdo his activities, causing pains and aches in the joints and muscles. In this case, you can seek the aid of aromatherapy blends. You can mix together 3 drops of lavender, 2 to 3 drops Copaiba, and a tablespoon of carrier oil then pour the mixture in a glass bottle with a roller ball.

   Anytime your dog shows signs of aching or sore muscles, you can just use the blend by rubbing its roller bottle into the affected area. Massage it gently, too. Expect him to obtain muscle ache relief within just ten to fifteen minutes.

With the three major recipes mentioned above and a couple of bonus recipes, it is safe to assume that aromatherapy for dogs can really help your furry friend live a healthy and happy life. Start taking full advantage of the power of aromatherapy as well as the beneficial and healing properties provided by the essential oils used in this technique to keep your dog at the pink of health.

What's good about aromatherapy is that it does not only work for dogs. You can also start researching about how you and your loved ones can benefit from it when it comes to boosting your health.

Thank you for taking the time to educate yourself before practicing the art of holistic medicine on your four legged pal. If you found this book helpful please remember to leave a review.

You may also want to check out my book of 100 essential oil recipes for dogs. Simply scan the QR code:

In addition to fully enjoying the benefits of holistic, non-intrusive healing, you can also take preventative measures by giving your best friend a healthy diet. Scan the QR code below to check out my dog food cookbook which includes 100 recipes that are easy and straight forward as well as guide to canine nutrition.

www.ingramcontent.com/pod-product-compliance
Lightning Source LLC
Chambersburg PA
CBHW070317230526
45470CB00002B/911